DEDICATION

I dedicate this book to my younger sister, Shelley. Bear in mind that even after giving birth, you can still be fit and get rid of that unwanted fats.

TABLE OF CONTENTS

Burn Fat and Become Fit With the Masters Fitness Guide

A Slimmer and Fat Free Body is Achieved

By: John Hamilton

9781634289856

PUBLISHERS NOTES

Disclaimer – Speedy Publishing LLC

This publication is intended to provide helpful and informative material. It is not intended to diagnose, treat, cure, or prevent any health problem or condition, nor is intended to replace the advice of a physician. No action should be taken solely on the contents of this book. Always consult your physician or qualified health-care professional on any matters regarding your health and before adopting any suggestions in this book or drawing inferences from it.

The author and publisher specifically disclaim all responsibility for any liability, loss or risk, personal or otherwise, which is incurred as a consequence, directly or indirectly, from the use or application of any contents of this book.

Any and all product names referenced within this book are the trademarks of their respective owners. None of these owners have sponsored, authorized, endorsed, or approved this book.

Always read all information provided by the manufacturers' product labels before using their products. The author and publisher are not responsible for claims made by manufacturers.

This book was originally printed before 2014. This is an adapted reprint by Speedy Publishing LLC with newly updated content designed to help readers with much more accurate and timely information and data.

Speedy Publishing LLC

40 E Main Street, Newark, Delaware, 19711

Contact Us: 1-888-248-4521

Website: http://www.speedypublishing.co

REPRINTED Paperback Edition: ISBN: 9781634289856

Manufactured in the United States of America

Chapter 1- Motivation to Burn that Fat

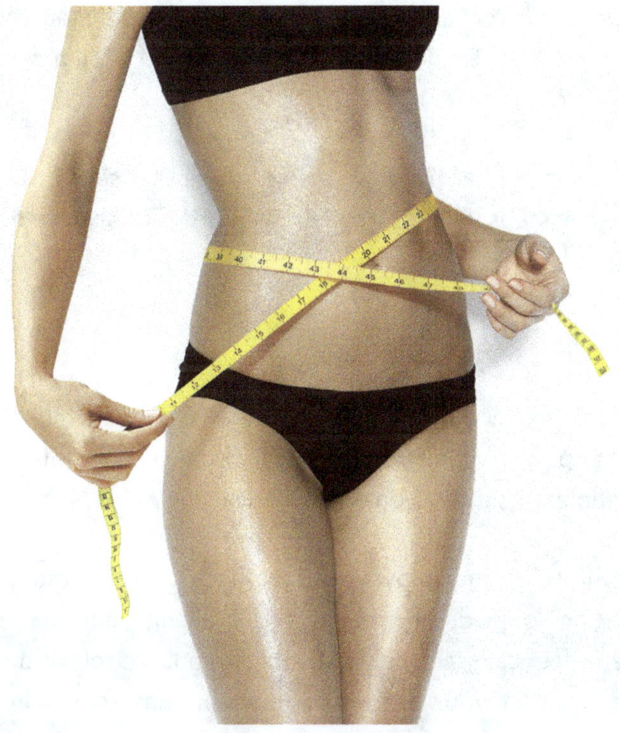

As you now know, the right mindset is crucial to gaining and maintaining that perfect weight and staying fat free forever. You need to learn and practice techniques that will enable you to stay enthusiastic and focused.

Visualization

One of the best techniques is visualization. Visualization is used by Olympic athletes, top business people and ordinary folk like you and me to mentally rehearse an outcome we desire.

This kind of mental rehearsal is incredibly powerful. By simply picturing the outcome you deeply and passionately desire you can literally make those thoughts come true. The trick, as ever, is to do it the right way.

Visualization works particularly well for fitness as the outcome you desire is so easy to picture. Try it – imagine a slimmer, toned version of yourself.

Now, was that so hard? OK, so it's not quite that simple. There are a number of steps you need to follow in order to achieve optimum results.

Visualization 1

This first exercise will teach you the basics while simultaneously achieving powerful results. It may seem simple but do not underestimate its effectiveness.

1. Sit comfortably and allow your breathing to slow without forcing it, taking in long, deep breaths and noticing your ribs expand. When you feel calm and relaxed, imagine a large television screen right in front of you. Picture yourself in that screen in bright, vibrant colors.

2. This picture of yourself is as you are now – above your ideal weight. Slowly imagine taking off your outer clothes so you are standing there in your underwear. Focus on your excess weight – go on, be brave and really examine it. Stare at your bulging belly. Take a good, hard look at your bulging hips and thighs.

3. Take note of your feelings about yourself. What are they? Acceptance? Disgust?

4. Now imagine the entire screen in front of you first of all fading until all the color has left it and then shrinking until it is the size of a postage stamp.

5. Begin to imagine another screen sliding in front of that postage stamp, growing bigger and bigger until it is the size of the old one.

6. Make this new screen even more vibrant and colorful than the last.

7. Imagine yourself in that screen, still in your underwear but now at your ideal weight.

8. How do you feel? Happy? Proud of yourself? Whatever positive feelings you get, intensify them. Actually feel them in your body. Smile.

9. Now squeeze one hand into a fist to allow your body to retain an imprinted memory of those feelings. Every time you waver in your exercise and nutritional program, repeat that same squeeze and those positive images and feelings will come flooding back to spur you on.

Visualization 2

This one is slightly more advanced and will be especially useful before you start exercising:

1. This time I want you to imagine the screen you created before actually inside your head.

2. Project an image of yourself as you are now on this screen but this time see yourself in your workout clothes.

3. Begin to imagine yourself exercising. Pick out a specific routine from the exercises detailed later on in this eBook. See yourself accomplishing this easily and successfully. ENJOY the exercise! Smile, relax. This is fun. This requires almost no effort. See yourself happy and accomplishing every movement with absolute ease.

4. Now imagine yourself standing tall after the exercise. See the beneficial results. See your stomach already flatter, your muscles leaner and stronger.

5. Repeat with another exercise. This time actually pull your stomach muscles in as you visualize and flex your arms and legs. This again will trigger muscle memory, matching up the positive images of you exercising and achieving great results with muscular movement.

6. Repeat one more time, each time getting leaner, fitter and stronger.

7. At first, do this before every exercise session. Even when you are well into the program and looking great, repeat this visualization every now and then to stoke up your motivation.

Self-Hypnosis

Self-hypnosis has become immensely popular among exercise professionals and for one very good reason: it works.

So what is self-hypnosis?

Think about all those times you've drifted off into a kind of trance or started to daydream. You may have done it while being totally absorbed in something like a book or a movie. You may even have done it when driving and then wondered how on earth you got to where you were going!

Although this same trance-like state of mind occurs during self-hypnosis the important difference is that you use that state to seed a specific motivation or goal in your brain.

Rather than the popular image of hypnosis as being something like sleep, it is actually a heightened state of awareness. The important thing is that, in this state, you suppress your critical faculties.

Take, for example, your desire to lose weight and keep it off. In your everyday state of mind you might have that thought or desire but that little, critical voice that pops up all too often for most of us will probably start telling you that it's impossible, that you don't deserve this, that you're never going to do it.

Using self-hypnosis means that we can turn that voice off. And once that voice is turned off we can plant positive suggestions much more successfully.

Just imagine how wonderful it must feel to be in a calm, peaceful state where you can convince yourself that anything is possible, that of course you can lose those extra pounds and, what's more, you can stay that way effortlessly.

Sounds good? Then let's do it!

First you have to ask yourself:

What do you want to achieve?

Self-hypnosis works best when you are clear and specific about your goals. It helps to write them down before you start as this can clarify them for you and make them seem more real.

In this case, you need to write down the ideal weight you want to achieve along with the measurements you are aiming to attain. Yes, that means stepping on those scales and getting out that tape measure but that's a good thing. Once you know what you're dealing with, you can set a realistic goal for you.

Once you have written down your goal, you need to:

Write out a plan

You need to plan what you are going to say and the best way to do this is to write yourself a mini script so that you can simply read off it without forgetting anything or stumbling over words.

Repeat your goals

Self hypnosis works best if you write out a number of suggestions for each goal you want to achieve. This will reinforce those suggestions deep into your subconscious in different ways and make it much more likely that your mind will accept the overall goal.

Some people prefer to speak into a digital recorder and then play back the result rather than simply talk themselves into a hypnotic state. This is fine so long as you make sure you keep your language and tone of voice as relevant to you as possible.

Create a vision of your success

Find or create some of your own images and symbols to represent and support your goal. Make this real so that they represent precisely how you wish to be. One great way to do this is to make a vision board, finding pictures of slim, healthful people and pasting them on a board so that you can refer to it often and certainly before your self-hypnosis session.

Personalize it

Always use your own words, i.e. the kind of language you would use everyday rather than something you feel you must say. Similarly, use images that appeal and are relevant to your lifestyle so that everything helps support your goal of becoming a better, slimmer you.

Think about suggestions that will really resonate with you. If you particularly hate your fat belly, you could say something like: 'My belly is already slimmer and, flatter thanks to my new routine and is going to carry on getting slimmer and flatter.'

Similarly, if you dislike the way you are always out of breath because you are overweight, tell yourself: 'I am now full of life and energy and have all the breath I need. Thanks to my new routine I become more energized every day.'

Use your own voice

If you are going to talk yourself down into a hypnotic state rather than use a recording then start your session in your normal voice and keep it nice and relaxed. Gradually start to slow as your session progresses, softening your voice so that you slip easily into a hypnotic state. Gradually return your voice to normal as you bring yourself out of your hypnotic state and back to reality.

Get comfortable

Always make sure your environment is as calm and peaceful as possible before you begin a self-hypnosis session. Never drive or operate any item of machinery while practicing self-hypnosis. You might like to use props such as soft music or low lighting but, for safety reasons, candles are not recommended.

Relaaaaaax

Start by sitting quietly and focusing internally, allowing your thoughts to just pass through your mind. Don't censor them or worry about anything – just let everything go and begin to breathe slowly and evenly.

Try, above all, not to judge yourself. You are about to implant new, positive messages in your mind that will enable you to not only reach your weight loss goal but to maintain your fat free self at a healthy weight forever!

Keep breathing and letting go of any anxieties or negativity. Be open to what is about to come and let any distractions simply float away from you.

Count yourself down

Start to imagine that you are descending a long staircase or floating down a stream to help yourself go deeper into a hypnotic state. Begin to count down in your mind at a slow and even pace, slipping into even more profound relaxation. Don't worry if your mind or body at first resists – simply keep counting and you will get there.

Arrive at your own special place

Once you are deeply relaxed, imagine yourself in the perfect environment. This is a place where you feel totally safe and where anything is possible. Make this is as vivid as possible. What can you see, hear and smell?

Once you feel comfortable, imagine yourself in this place only this you is already slimmer and healthier. Begin to implant the suggestions you already planned or simply listen to them if you are using a recording. Allow them to sink in but, again, don't judge or criticize them or yourself in any way.

Set yourself up for next time

Once you have absorbed all those positive, powerful messages include some suggestions to help you when you come out of your trance. You could use something like: 'After this session I will feel twice as motivated and am already looking forward to the next one.'

Count yourself back

At the end of your session, count yourself back to full awareness. Suggest to yourself that when you leave hypnosis you will feel refreshed and alert. Check that you are once again fully awake and alert and enjoy the rest of your day!

CHAPTER 2- BURN FAT AND BECOME FIT WITH FAT FREE FOOD

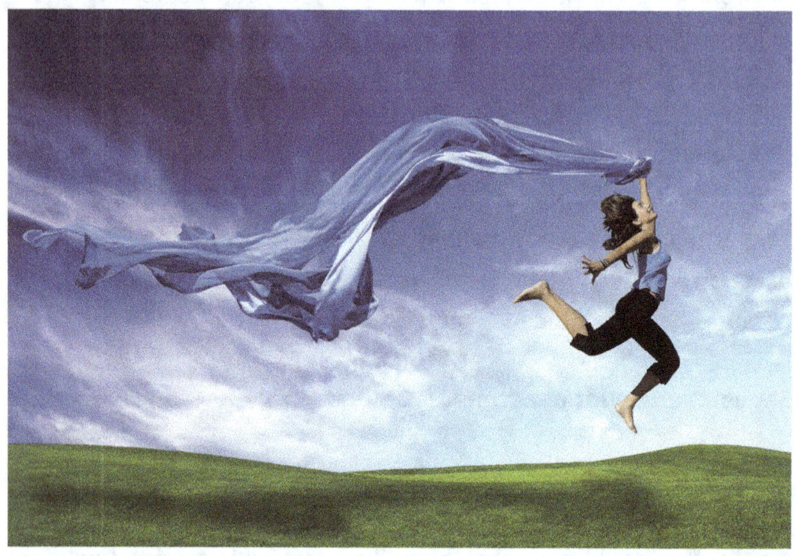

Anyone who has ever tried to diet knows that sooner or later you get bored. It's inevitable when your choices are restricted. I therefore want you to look on this section as a re-education rather than a diet. Once you know what and how to eat you will find that the possibilities are endless.

It's also important that you understand that attitude is as important when applied to food as it is to exercise. Too many of us are brought up with or acquire unhealthy notions of what food represents.

We hear and read all kinds of things – that certain foods are 'bad' or 'fattening.' Of course there are foods that contain little if any nutritional value and these are to be avoided but no one food group is inherently bad or fattening provided it is ingested as part of a balanced diet.

Take fat, for example. For many people it's a huge no no. They buy all kinds of low-fat products, unaware that they are actually doing their bodies more harm than good.

Those low-fat products may plaster all kinds of fancy claims on their packaging but read the label closely (and this is something I encourage you always do when shopping) and you will find that what is left out in fat is made up for in increased sugar, salt and chemicals.

As human beings we need fat. It's the densest form of calorific energy we can ingest. The trick is to choose the right kind of fat and that's simple: keep it as natural as possible.

I would rather eat butter any day than the highly processed, hydrogenated polyunsaturated fats prevalent in so many supposedly 'healthy' or 'diet' products. The crucial factor here is that I eat moderate amounts of butter. Rather than slather it on my toast I simply scrape on a small amount.

The same goes for oils. By preference, I'll pick a good olive oil over almost any other both to cook with and to dress salads. You will never find one of those revolting 'diet' dressings in my cupboards because I refuse to feed my body with what is essentially a cocktail of chemicals.

If you don't believe me, read the label. Do you really want to eat a whole bunch of artificial additives and preservatives, some of which may be linked with serious diseases including cancer?

And here's the thing: these additives and preservatives can also cause bloating. So while you are doing your innocent best to slim down, you are actually making yourself look and feel fatter.

Burn Fat and Become Fit With the Masters Fitness Guide

The truth is that no natural fat is bad for you provided you follow the 20-40 rules. Keep your fat intake to this percentage of your diet, ensure that it is part of a balanced, healthy eating plan and you will be able to enjoy all kinds of foods while actually losing weight.

Aside from examples such as butter and oil, there are other healthy sources of fat. These include nuts, seeds and avocadoes – all things you may have previously considered to be 'fattening' or unhealthy.

Again, the key is moderation. A handful of Brazil nuts rather than a bowl of salted peanuts, for example. A snack of seeds rather than a low quality chocolate bar full of poor grade hydrogenated fats and sugar.

As for chocolate, that's another thing you can indulge in now and then provided it is at least 70% cocoa solids and the best quality you can afford. This type of chocolate contains less sugar and milk chocolate and will also satisfy your taste buds far more, meaning that you will automatically eat less as you savor it rather than simply gobbling it up.

Fancy a glass of wine? Have it. Just make sure it's a small glass and that you buy organic if at all possible. The same goes for red meat and poultry – eat less of the best you can afford.

Organic, grass-fed beef will be far leaner than the mass produced stuff packed full of hormones. Free range chicken may be more expensive but you will actually receive more for your money as it will not have been injected with water and chemicals to plump it up.

There is strong evidence that the simpler and cleaner we keep our diets the healthier and leaner we become. Another top tip is to only eat what is in season, thereby lessening the chance of your food having been artificially produced and then kept fresh for shipping with quantities of artificial additives.

On the following pages you will find suggestions for healthy sources of fat, carbohydrate and protein. Use these lists in conjunction with the healthy eating sample plans and you will be more than halfway to becoming and remaining fat free forever.

Chapter 3- Food Sources to Burn Fat and Become Fit

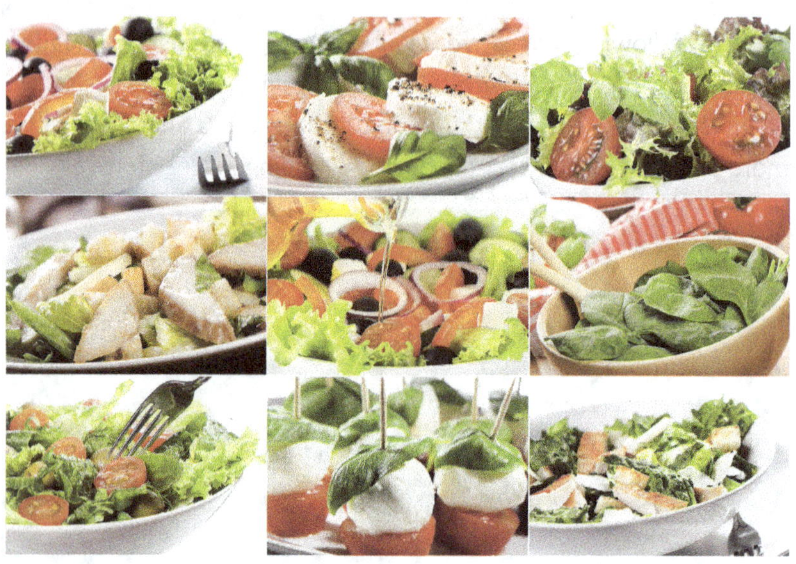

Healthy Sources of Carbohydrate

Butter

Olive oil – especially cold-pressed, extra virgin

Sunflower oil

Other unrefined vegetable oils

Fish oil

Nuts

Seeds

Fruits Whole grain cereals

Vegetables Whole grain pasta

Beans some dairy products

Nuts

Legumes

Whole grain breads

Healthy Sources of Protein

Organic, grass-fed red meat Unrefined dairy products

Free-range chicken Beans

Duck Nuts

Goose Pulses

Fish – preferably not farmed Eggs

Shellfish Soy (miso and tempeh)

Keeping The GI Low

As well as choosing healthy foods from the previous tables, you also need to be aware of the Glycemic Index (or GI) of those foods so your choice can be even more informed.

The GI score for each food will tell you the rate at which the sugar in that food will be absorbed. The quicker the GI score, the faster the sugar is absorbed.

The lower the score, the better for you as it will mean sustained, slow release energy that is far less likely to cause stomach bloating or lethargy.

Eating Right

To kick start your routine and get you seeing results fast, I recommend a four day plan that will help introduce your body to healthy eating. The reward for this will be a metabolism that is speeded up rather than slowed down by traditional 'diet' plans.

First off, for these initial four days you are going to be eating six small meals a day. It has been proven that such an eating pattern helps initiate weight loss by keeping your metabolism working at a consistently high level.

You will be basing these meals on foods high in healthy monounsaturated fats as well as fruits, vegetables and fiber-rich whole grains, all designed to make sure you feel full.

4 Day Kick-Start

Day One

Breakfast

Small bowl natural probiotic yoghurt mixed with 1 teaspoon honey. Substitute with soy yoghurt if necessary.

1 small pear or apple

3 or 4 Brazil nuts

Herbal tea or unsweetened juice

Lunch

2 slices organic chicken/hard cheese

Small mixed salad scattered with sunflower seeds

Water or herbal tea

Snack smoothie (see recipe)

Dinner

Grilled white fish with handful of mange tout or green beans, 2 or 3 new steamed potatoes drizzled with 1tsp olive oil

Water or herbal tea

Day Two

Breakfast

Small bowl wholegrain, unsweetened cereal with skimmed milk (preferably goat – substitute soy or nut milk as necessary)

4 walnuts

200g melon cubed or sliced

Herbal tea or unsweetened juice

Lunch

Tuna salad made with small tin of tuna in spring water, 2 tbsp natural yoghurt, diced cucumber, tomato and shredded lettuce all mixed together

2 whole-wheat crackers or crisp breads

Water or herbal tea

Snack smoothie (see recipe below)

Dinner

Chicken stroganoff made with small chicken breast, small onion, and 1 clove garlic and button mushrooms sautéed in 1tsp olive oil with 1 teaspoon paprika. Stir in two tablespoons natural yoghurt and serve with a handful of cooked brown rice

Water or herbal tea

Day Three

Breakfast

2 slices rye bread toasted and spread thinly with butter and 1 tsp honey

Handful of mixed seeds

1 apple or pear

Herbal tea or unsweetened juice

Lunch

1 bowl vegetable or chicken broth

2 slices hard cheese

2 whole-wheat crackers or crisp breads

Water or herbal tea

Snack smoothie (see recipe below)

Dinner

1 grilled salmon fillet served with mange tout or green beans and 1 small potato thinly sliced and sautéed in 1tsp olive oil

Water or herbal tea

Day Four

Breakfast

1 small bowl of porridge served with skimmed milk and 1 tsp honey if liked. Substitute with wholegrain cereal if you dislike porridge.

1 apple or pear

Herbal tea or unsweetened juice

Lunch

Small bowl of whole-wheat pasta, cooked and then dressed with 1 tbsp olive oil, black pepper and 50g grated hard cheese

1 small mixed salad

1 mango or peach

Water or herbal tea

Snack smoothie (recipe below)

Dinner

1 grilled chicken breast marinated in 1 tsp of soy sauce mixed with 1 tsp honey and served with 1 small, sliced zucchini and 2 or 3 mushrooms sautéed with 1tsp olive oil.

Serve with handful of cooked brown rice

Water or herbal tea

Smoothie Recipes

Apricot, Pineapple & Strawberry Smoothie

1/4 cup crushed pineapple, canned or fresh

1 fresh apricot, diced, seed removed

6 strawberries, frozen

1/2 banana, cut in chunks, frozen

1 1/2 cup water

1 tbsp. skim milk powder

In a blender, process fruit with the rest of the ingredients. Blend until thoroughly mixed and serve.

Banana & Strawberry Smoothie

1 banana, cut in chunks, frozen

6 strawberries, frozen

1 1/4 cup water

1 tbsp. skim milk powder

In a blender, process all the ingredients until thoroughly mixed and serve.

Tropical Smoothie

1/2 mango, peeled, seed removed

1/8 tsp. natural coconut extract

1/2 banana, cut in chunks, frozen

4 strawberries, frozen

6 ice cubes

1 1/4 cups water

In a blender, process all the ingredients until thoroughly mixed and serve.

Banana Berry Smoothie

1/2 banana, cut in chunks, frozen

1/2 pear, cored and sliced

1/4 cup frozen blueberries

1 1/4 cup water

1 tbsp. skim milk powder

1/8 tsp. cinnamon

In a blender, process all the ingredients until thoroughly mixed and serve.

Banana, Orange & Strawberry Smoothie

1/2 banana, cut in chunks, frozen

6 strawberries, frozen

1/2 cup orange juice

1/2 cup water

1 tbsp. skim milk powder

In a blender, process all the ingredients until thoroughly blended and serve.

Banana, Palm Sugar & Apple Smoothie

1 ripe banana, peeled and halved

150 ml natural yoghurt

1 teaspoon palm sugar or honey

1 apple

200 ml skimmed milk or soy milk

In a blender, process all the ingredients until thoroughly blended and serve.

Mango & Orange Smoothie

1 small, ripe mango, peeled and sliced

2 oranges, juiced

Half a lime or lemon, juiced

2 ice cubes

In a blender, process all the ingredients until thoroughly blended and serve.

Peach, Pear & Raspberry Smoothie

1 ripe peach, peeled and sliced

1 ripe pear, peeled, cored and sliced

3 raspberries

2 tbsp yoghurt

1 teaspoon runny honey

2 ice cubes

Put ice and yoghurt in blender and blend for a few seconds until ice is crushed. Still blending, add peach slices then pear. Finally, add raspberries one by one and honey if liked. Blend until smooth.

Rhubarb & Ginger Smoothie

2 stems rhubarb

1 orange

1 teaspoon runny honey

Little grated, fresh ginger

2 ice cubes

Squeeze the juice from the oranges and place in a small pan with the rhubarb, honey, ginger and 1 or 2 tablespoons water. Stir over medium heat until sugar dissolves then cover pan and stew rhubarb over low heat until it softens, adding more water if necessary. Let it cool. Put ice cubes in blender and blend for a few seconds. Add rhubarb mixture and blend until smooth. Drink immediately.

Eating Right – Next Steps

Below you will find suggestions for meal plans suitable for various body types. Remember that these are just suggestions and that you can mix and match sensibly and within reason.

Snacks:

Pick 2 snacks a day from the following list and eat one mid-morning and one mid-afternoon:

1 hardboiled egg

1/2 orange

Sprinkled w/ peanuts

1/2 cup plain yogurt

Sprinkled w/ pecans

1 oz cheese

1/2 apple

1 macadamia nut

1 oz canned chicken or tuna

1 peach

1/2 tsp peanut butter

1 1/2 oz deli-style ham or turkey

1 carrot

5 olives

1 oz mozzarella string cheese

1/2 cup grapes

1 Tbs avocado

1 oz jack cheese

1 Tbs guacamole

1 tomato

1 oz hummus

1/2 tomato

1 1/2 oz feta cheese

1 cup strawberries

1/4 cup cottage cheese

1 macadamia nut

1 poached egg

1/2 slice bread

1/2 tsp peanut butter

1/4 cup cottage cheese

1/2 carrot

3 celery stalks

5 olives

3 oz marinated and baked tofu

1/2 apple

1/2 tsp peanut butter

1 oz tuna

1 large tossed salad

1 tsp salad dressing of choice

1 hardboiled egg

1 large spinach salad

1 tsp oil and vinegar dressing

1 oz grilled turkey breast

1/2 cup blueberries

3 cashews

1/4 cup cottage cheese

1 cup sliced tomato

1/3 tsp olive oil

1 1/2 oz deli-style turkey

1 tangerine

1 Tbs avocado

1 1/2 oz shrimp

2 cups broccoli

6 peanuts

1 1/2 oz feta cheese

1 cup diced tomato

5 olives

1 oz sardines

1/2 nectarine

5 olives

1 oz cheddar cheese melted over

1/2 apple

Sprinkled w/ walnuts

1 1/2 oz scallops

1 sliced cucumber

1/2 tsp tartar sauce

Remember, these eating plans are guidelines. Follow them for at least two weeks after your 4 day kick-start program and then use the healthy recipes in the next section to maintain your new slender frame.

Healthy Recipes

You can mix and match these recipes to maintain your healthy weight. It is important, however, to stick to the ratio of quantities suggested and not to add unhealthy ingredients such as extra oil or sugar.

Whole-Wheat Spaghetti with Swiss Chard and Pecorino Cheese

Ingredients

1 tablespoon olive oil

2 onions, thinly sliced

2 bunches Swiss chard, trimmed and chopped (about 14 cups)

3 garlic cloves, minced

1 (14 1/2-ounce) can diced tomatoes with juices

1/4 cup dry white wine

1/4 teaspoon dried crushed red pepper flakes

Salt and pepper

8 ounces whole-wheat spaghetti

1/4 cup pitted kalamata olives, coarsely chopped

2 tablespoons freshly grated Pecorino cheese

2 tablespoons toasted pine nuts

Directions

Heat the oil in a heavy large frying pan over medium heat. Add the onions and sauté until tender, about 8 minutes. Add the chard and sauté until it wilts, about 2 minutes. Add the garlic and sauté until fragrant, about 1 minute. Stir in the tomatoes with their juices, wine, and red pepper flakes. Bring to a simmer. Cover and simmer until the tomatoes begin to break down and the chard is very tender, stirring occasionally, about 5 minutes. Season the chard mixture, to taste, with salt and pepper.

Meanwhile, bring a large pot of salted water to a boil. Add the spaghetti and cook until tender but still firm to the bite, stirring frequently, about 8 to 10 minutes. Drain the spaghetti. Add the spaghetti to the chard mixture and toss to combine.

Transfer the pasta to serving bowls. Sprinkle the olives, cheese, and pine nuts and serve.

Serves 4.

Bruschetta with White Beans, Sun-dried Tomatoes and Basil

Ingredients - For the Beans

3/4 cup cannelloni beans

1/4 cup extra-virgin olive oil

1 garlic clove, peeled

1 bay leaf

1/2 teaspoon salt

Ingredients - For the bruschetta and topping

1 small baguette, sliced into thick pieces

1 tablespoon thinly sliced garlic, plus 1 garlic clove, peeled, for coating bread

2 tablespoons extra-virgin olive oil

1/2 teaspoon chili flakes

8 to 10 basil leaves

1/3 cup oil-packed sun-dried tomatoes, drained and sliced

1/4-inch thick

2 tablespoons chopped fresh parsley

Lemon juice

Salt and fresh black pepper

2 ounces ricotta salata cheese, grated large

Directions

Beans

Rinse the beans well and then put in a 1-quart saucepan. Cover with water to 1-inch over the top of the beans. On medium-high heat, bring to a boil. Immediately take the pot away from the burner, cover and hold for 1 hour. Change the water; add half of the extra-virgin olive oil, 1 garlic clove and the bay leaf. Cook beans on low. Simmer for about 40 minutes or until tender. During last 10 minutes, add 1/2 teaspoon salt. Stir in carefully. Remove from heat and hold in the saucepan with the cooking liquid until cool. This may be done 1 to 2 days before serving, and kept refrigerated.

Bruschetta Topping

Preheat a grill or stove-top grill pan.

Grill the bread on both sides until crispy. Be careful on high heat as bread burns easily.

While bread is grilling, in a sauté pan on medium heat, toast the sliced garlic in the olive oil. When it is light golden, add the chili flakes, cook for 10 seconds and then add the basil leaves. Do this carefully, as the basil may spatter some oil.

With a slotted spoon, transfer the beans to the pan. Add 1 to 2 tablespoons of the bean cooking liquid (or liquid from canned beans) and mix all together. Hold warm. Adjust consistency, as necessary, with the bean liquid, a little at a time.

When the basil leaves are wilted, remove mixture from the heat. Add the sun-dried tomatoes and chopped parsley. Toss to combine and adjust the seasoning with lemon juice, to taste, and salt and pepper.

Lightly swipe the remaining garlic clove on 1 side of the bread. Arrange the toasted bruschetta on a serving platter and drizzle with the remaining extra-virgin olive oil. Top each piece with some of the tomato-bean mixture, then evenly divide the ricotta salata over the mixture. Serve warm.

Serves 3.

Three Bean and Beef Chili

Ingredients

1 tablespoon olive oil

1 onion, diced (1 cup)

1 red bell pepper, diced (1 cup)

2 carrots, diced (1/2 cup)

2 teaspoons ground cumin

1 pound extra-lean ground beef (90 percent lean)

1 (28-ounce) can crushed tomatoes

2 cups water

1 chipotle chile in adobo sauce, seeded and minced

2 teaspoons adobo sauce from the can of chipotles

1/2 teaspoon dried oregano

Salt and freshly ground black pepper

1 (15.5-ounce) can black beans, drained and rinsed

1 (15.5-ounce) can kidney beans, drained and rinsed

1 (15.5-ounce) can pinto beans, drained and rinsed

Directions

Heat the oil in large pot or Dutch oven over moderate heat. Add the onion, bell pepper and carrots, cover and cook, stirring occasionally until the vegetables are soft, about 10 minutes. Add the cumin and cook, stirring, for 1 minute. Add the ground beef; raise the heat to high and cook, breaking up the meat with a spoon, until the meat is no longer pink. Stir in the tomatoes, water, chipotle and adobo sauce, oregano and salt and pepper. Cook, partially covered, stirring from time to time, for 30 minutes. Stir in the beans and continue cooking, partially covered, 20 minutes longer. Season, to taste, with salt and pepper.

Serves 8, serving size 1 1/4 cup.

Salmon with Lemon, Capers, and Rosemary

Ingredients

4 (6-ounce) salmon fillets

1/4 cup extra-virgin olive oil

1/2 teaspoon salt

1/2 teaspoon freshly ground black pepper

1 tablespoon minced fresh rosemary leaves

8 lemon slices (about 2 lemons)

1/4 cup lemon juice (about 1 lemon)

1/2 cup Marsala wine (or white wine)

4 teaspoons capers

4 pieces of aluminum foil

Directions

Brush top and bottom of salmon fillets with olive oil and season with salt, pepper, and rosemary. Place each piece of seasoned salmon on a piece of foil large enough to fold over and seal. Top the each piece of salmon with 2 lemon slices, 1 tablespoon of lemon juice, 2 tablespoons of wine, and 1 teaspoon of capers. Wrap up salmon tightly in the foil packets.

Place a grill pan over medium-high heat or preheat a gas or charcoal grill. Place the foil packets on the hot grill and cook for 10 minutes for a 1-inch thick piece of salmon. Serve in the foil packets.

Serves 4.

Chicken Piccata with Pasta and Mushrooms

Ingredients

6 ounces whole-wheat angel hair pasta

1/3 cup all-purpose flour, divided

2 cups reduced-sodium chicken broth

1/2 teaspoon salt, divided

1/4 teaspoon freshly ground pepper

4 chicken cutlets (3/4-1 pound total), trimmed

3 teaspoons extra-virgin olive oil, divided

1 10-ounce package mushrooms, sliced

3 large cloves garlic, minced

1/2 cup white wine

2 tablespoons lemon juice

1/4 cup chopped fresh parsley

2 tablespoons capers, rinsed

2 teaspoons butter

Directions

Bring a large pot of water to a boil. Add pasta and cook until just tender, 4 to 6 minutes or according to package directions. Drain and rinse.

Meanwhile, whisk 5 teaspoons flour and broth in a small bowl until smooth. Place the remaining flour in a shallow dish. Season chicken with 1/4 teaspoon salt and pepper and dredge both sides in the flour. Heat 2 teaspoons oil in a large non-stick skillet over medium heat. Add the chicken and cook until browned and no longer pink in the middle, 2 to 3 minutes per side. Transfer to a plate; keep warm.

Heat the remaining 1 teaspoon oil in the pan over medium-high heat. Add mushrooms and cook, stirring, until they release their juices and begin to brown, about 5 minutes. Transfer to a plate. Add garlic and wine to the pan and cook until reduced by half, 1 to 2 minutes. Stir in the reserved broth-flour mixture, lemon juice and the remaining 1/4 teaspoon salt. Bring to a simmer and cook, stirring, until the sauce is thickened, about 5 minutes.

Stir in parsley, capers, butter and the reserved mushrooms. Measure out 1/2 cup of the mushroom sauce. Toss the pasta in the pan with the remaining sauce. Serve the pasta topped with the chicken and the reserved sauce.

Serves 4.

Chick Pea Salad

Salads made with lots of beans are healthy and full of fiber. This salad can be made with chickpeas, black beans, kidney beans, or black-eyed peas—they're all delicious.

Ingredients

Water for blanching 1 cup broccoli florets 1 15-oz. can chickpeas (garbanzo beans), drained 1 tomato, diced 1 stalk celery, sliced 1/4 cup low fat/fat free mayonnaise or salad dressing 2 Tbsp. lemon juice 1 clove garlic, minced 1 Tbsp. minced fresh parsley 1 Tbsp. chopped onion Pepper, to taste

Directions

Bring the water to a boil. Add the broccoli and cook for about 2 minutes, then transfer to a colander and immediately run under cold water to stop the cooking process.

In a medium bowl, mix all the ingredients until just combined

Serve over lettuce.

Serves 2 as a meal and 4 as a side dish

Pizza Bianca

Ingredients

Readymade pizza crust 1/8 cup extra-virgin olive oil 5 cloves garlic, minced 1 16 ounce pkg. shredded, reduced fat mozzarella cheese 1/4 cup sliced onion 1/4 cup sliced kalamata olives 1/4 cup quartered canned or bottled artichoke hearts, drained Pepper, to taste

Directions

Combine the olive oil with the garlic and let sit for about 15 minutes.

Place pizza shell on a pizza pan or baking sheet.

Top with the olive oil and garlic mixture.

Sprinkle the cheese onto the pizza.

Top with the onions, olives, and artichokes.

Bake at 450°F for 10 minutes or until edge of crust is browned and cheese is melted.

Makes 1 pizza

Dulce De Leche Fingers

Ingredients

4 Fajita size soft flour tortillas (34 grams)

4 tablespoons of dulce de leche

1 ounce of sliced almonds

1 large red delicious apple (10 ounces) sliced and divided in four portions

Directions

Spread 1 tablespoon of dulce de leche on a flour tortilla.

Sprinkle ¼ ounce of sliced almonds evenly over the tortilla.

Take ¼ of sliced apple and lay the pieces 2 inches from the edge of the tortilla.

Fold the tortilla covering the sliced apples and roll.

Repeat with remaining tortillas.

Place tortilla fingers in microwave for 10 seconds.

Serves 4.

Cinnamon Caramel Bananas

Ingredients

4 Bananas

2 tsp Brown sugar

1/2 tsp Vanilla

1/4 tsp Cinnamon

1/2 tablespoon Butter

Vanilla ice cream

Graham crackers

Caramel sauce

Directions

Separate ingredients into 2 bowls.

Slice bananas, top with the rest of the ingredients.

Microwave for about 20-30 seconds, stir.

Serve with Ice Cream, crushed up graham crackers and caramel sauce.

Serves 4.

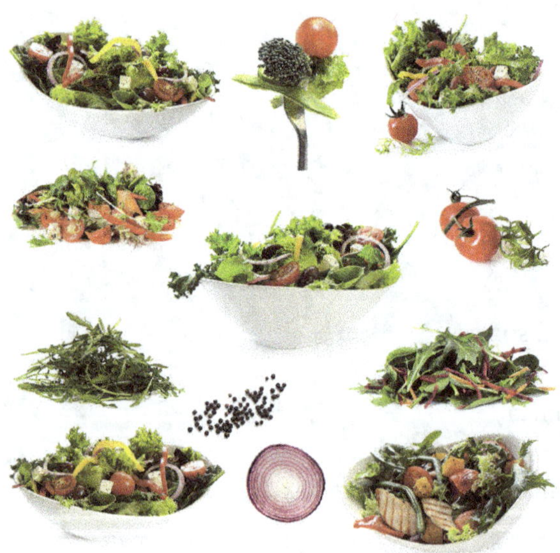

Chapter 4- Burn Fat and Become Fit Workout

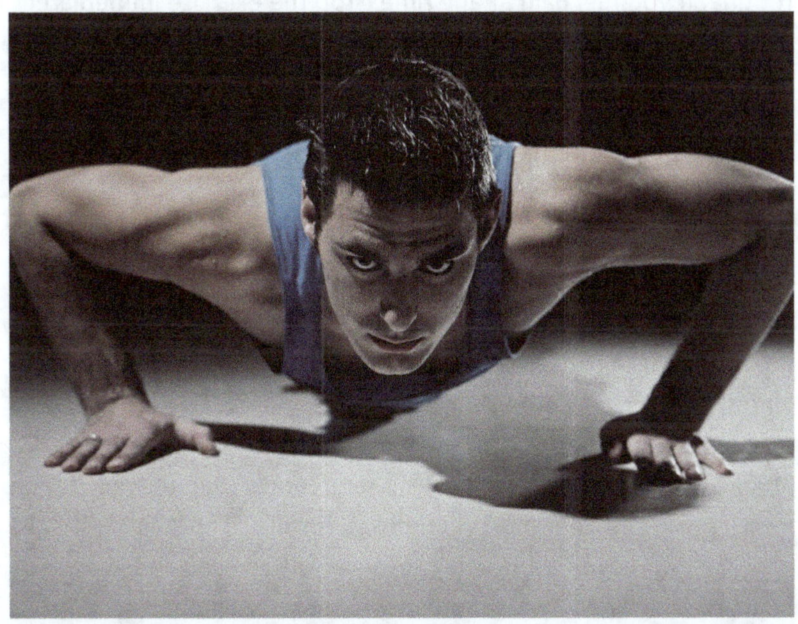

It is a myth that, in order to burn fat, you need to subject yourself to hours of boring cardio-based exercise. In fact, strength training combined with interval training produces optimum results.

The good news about this is that you can achieve a lot in a short space of time. Even better, you start to see a result fast which in turn motivates you to keep going.

A combination of strength and interval training will force your body to burn carbohydrate to supply it with the necessary energy. The right kind of carbohydrate, low GI, is supplied when you follow the nutritional guidelines in this book. Using the exercise and eating tactics in this book synergistically, therefore, will guarantee success.

The following exercises are suitable for all ages and both sexes. If you are pregnant or suffer from any kind of chronic or recurring injury, consult a medical practitioner before beginning any exercise routine. If you feel pain at any time, stop the exercise immediately, rest and seek advice if appropriate. Remember to follow the instructions carefully for a safe, highly effective workout.

Get Your Heart Pumping

Yes, I know I promised no hours of boring cardio and here I am going to keep my promise. How? By encouraging you to undertake exercise you actually enjoy and to then suggest you reinforce that enjoyment using the NLP techniques such as Anchoring that you learned earlier.

Studies have shown that exercising for at least 30 minutes 5 days a week produces the most beneficial results. The thing is, that exercise can cover a huge range of activities provided that your heart rate is raised to a suitable level for your age and remains at that level for the majority of the exercise period.

Working Out Your Heart Rate

To find your working heart rate, or the optimal level at which you should be exercising, you first need to work out your resting heart rate which will give you a good indication of how your fitness is improving.

The best way to do this is to check your pulse for 60 seconds before you get out of bed in the morning. The fitter you get, the lower this will become.

So What Sort Of Cardio Exercise Should I Do?

This is the fun part – almost anything provided it is safe and follows the criteria for raising your heart rate. I like to mix it up, one day alternating fast walking with jogging in the park, another attending a folk dance class and so on.

The simplest routine is one that is also highly effective – just going for a power walk, arms pumping at sufficient pace will provide a low impact route to stripping excess fat from your body.

Remember, however, what you learned in the sections on motivation.

It's crucial to keep boredom at bay and to constantly push yourself just that little bit more.

For these reasons, I advocate a class or new hobby that is both physical and fun. Some ideas include:

- Tennis
- Cycling
- Soccer
- Volleyball
- Hiking
- Dancing of all types
- Boxing
- Canoeing
- Rowing
- Skiing
- Water-skiing
- Wind-surfing
- Surfing

The possibilities are literally endless and half the joy comes from mastering a new skill which, in turn, boosts your new found confidence.

Ideally, you would split your exercise routine into four or five sessions with one or two devoted to your new hobby or sport and the others mixing up cardio with the routines outlined below.

Of course, there are times when this is not possible due to constraints of work or family, for example, and this is where keeping it simple will also keep you on track.

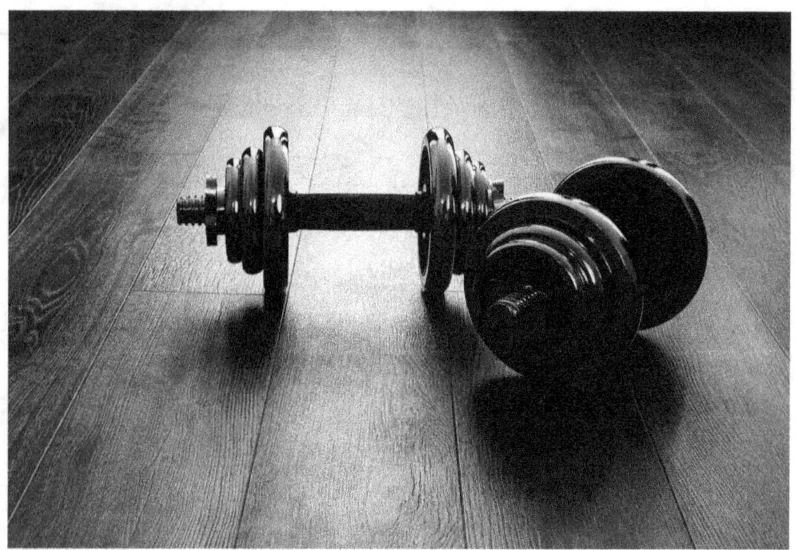

Chapter 5- Healthy Cooking Tips to Burn Fat & Become Fit

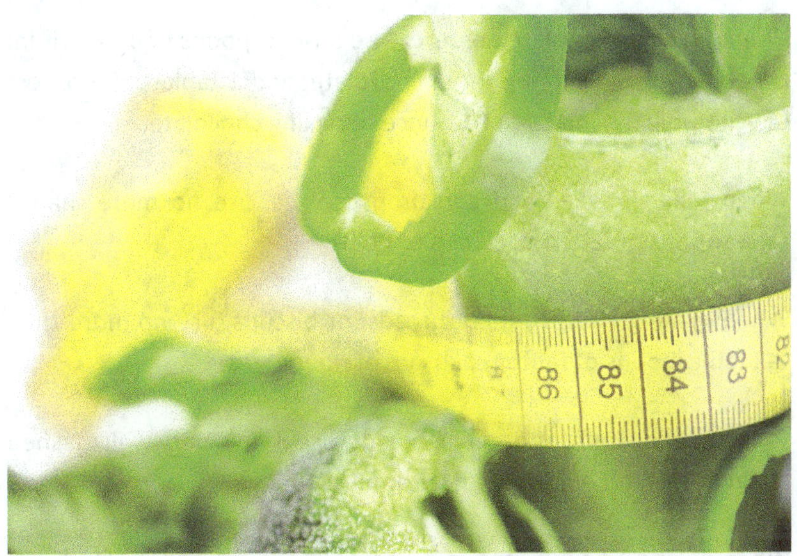

Try this when cooking potatoes: Rather than home fries in butter, layer sliced potatoes (with some onion slices) in a cast iron skillet coated with no stick spray. Brush tops lightly with vegetable oil. Sprinkle with paprika and freshly cracked pepper. Roast the potatoes in the skillet in a 425 degree oven for 20 to 30 minutes or until potatoes are brown on top.

To de-fat homemade broths, soups and stew, prepare the food ahead and chill it. Before reheating the food, lift off the hardened fat formed at the surface. Or, if you don't have the time to chill the food, float a few ice cubes on the surface of the warm liquid to harden the fat. Then remove the fat and discard.

When sautéing onion for flavoring stews, soups and sauces, use non-stick spray, water or stock.

When making a salad dressing, use equal parts water and vinegar and half as much oil. To make up for less intense flavor, add more mustard and herbs.

When making chocolate desserts, use 3 tablespoons of cocoa (if fat is needed to replace the fat in chocolate, add 1 tablespoon or less of vegetable oil) instead of 1 ounce of baking chocolate.

When making cakes and soft-drop cookies, use no more than 2 tablespoons of fat for each cup of flour.

When making muffins, quick breads, or biscuits, use no more than 1-2 tablespoons of fat for each cup of flour.

When making muffins or quick breads, use 3 ripe, very well mashed bananas instead of ½ cup butter or oil.

When baking or cooking, use 3 egg whites and 1 yolk instead of 2 whole eggs; use 2 egg whites instead of 1 whole egg.

When making pie crust, use only ½ cup margarine for every 2 cups of flour.

When you need sour cream, blend 1 cup low fat cottage cheese with 1 tablespoon skim milk and 2 tablespoons lemon juice, substitute plain or nonfat/low fat yogurt, or try some of the reduced fat sour cream substitutes.

Use non-stick vegetable sprays instead of butter.

Use oil instead of shortening, butter, or margarine.

Substitute vegetables or beans for meat, poultry or fish in recipes.

Season your meals with herbs and spices instead of salt.

Lemon juice is also a great low-sodium seasoning.

You can cut the sugar in baked goods down by ¼ or ½, but you cannot do this for cakes or yeast breads.

Read the labels of canned fruits, and look for ones that have been packed in their own juices.

Add vanilla or cinnamon when sugar has been cut to keep foods sweet and interesting.

Replace half of the white flour with whole wheat flour.

Use brown rice instead of white rice.

Add oatmeal or other whole grains to breads.

Add fruits for a sweet treat.

Add more vegetables to your favorite dishes.

CHAPTER 6- BURN FAT & BECOME FIT – POST PREGNANCY PROBLEM

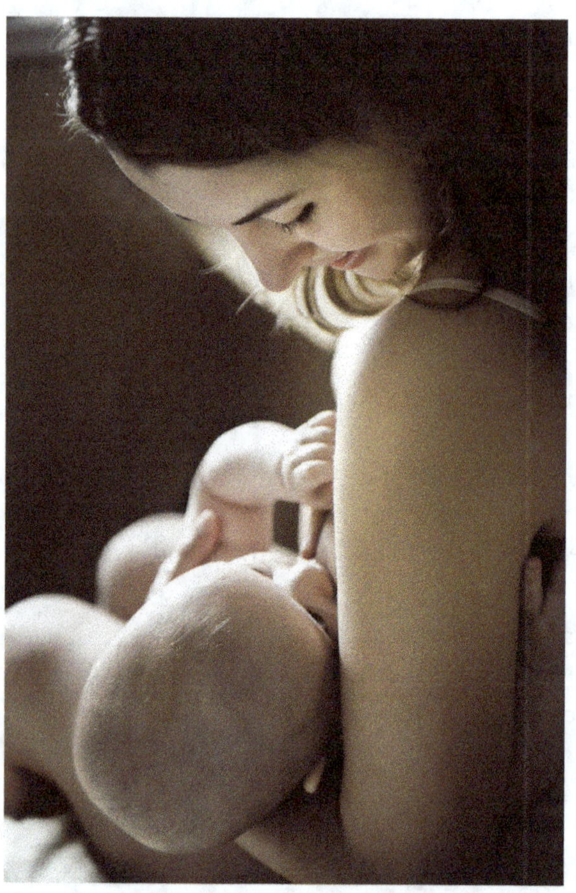

Breastfeeding

Many women who have recently given birth are always interested in attempting to lose some of that extra weight that traditionally accompanies having a baby. What many of these women do not entirely realize is the fact that breast-feeding can not only help provide the baby with essential vitamins and nutrients, but can also help in the weight-loss process.

For example, the average mother will utilize somewhere between 500 calories and 800 calories a day producing milk for the baby. Not only will the baby receive the health and nutrition that it needs, but it may also enable a woman to lose baby fat a lot faster.

As you can probably already imagine, it is a lot easier to say that going to the gym and cutting back on the amount of food that one need is the easiest path to losing weight. That being said, it's not really a practical option for many new mothers. There are a lot of responsibilities associated with having a baby which require a great deal of focus and effort.

There's certainly nothing wrong with trying to eat healthy food and attempting to engage in some type of exercise on a regular basis. However, the point is that breast-feeding can really augment a new mother effort to lose weight. Remember, as mentioned a moment ago, between 500 calories in 800 calories a day are often consumed in the process of creating the milk that will be fed to the baby.

Something that a lot of new mothers often times do is try to interact with other new mothers who find themselves dealing with a variety of similar challenges. One of those challenges is losing some of the extra weight that is acquired as a result of the pregnancy. Women often times find it a lot easier to lose weight when they are able to communicate their peers and anxieties with other women and to support each other as they go about the process of shedding the extra pounds put on during pregnancy.

In this regard, breast-feeding is a wonderful tool because he really doesn't require any extra effort. It's just something that naturally happens. In addition to breast-feeding, taking walks and making an effort to eat low-fat food can really start to make a difference. As always, if in doubt, speak your doctor to make sure that you are doing what is best for your health as well as that of your new baby.

2.Drink Plenty Of Water

Drinking plenty of water is something else that can dramatically help a new mother lose weight. How is this possible? And to be realistic, how much weight can actually be lost using this method? Let's dig into this issue.

The very first thing you need to understand is that water has no calories whatsoever. We are not talking about special water that you might buy at a grocery store that contains sugar or other additives which contain calories. The water we are referring to is the basic water they can come right from the tap.

You may be wondering why it is significant that water has no calories. When you stop and think about it, we all need to drink something. Why drink a beverage that contains calories if your goal is to lose baby fat ? Most medical studies have strongly suggested that the overwhelming majority of people will get all the hydration that they need from water. You don't need to drink sugary sodas to become hydrated.

This raises the question of whether or not diet soda is a suitable alternative to water. After all, the amount of calories contained in diet soda can be extremely low. What you need to remember is that a lot of scientists have concluded that your body performs better and is less likely to develop problems related to excess weight when you drink water. In addition, there are a lot of artificial sweeteners that are used in various types of soft drinks. This could have a negative impact on your baby assuming that you are breast-feeding.

Drinking water is not enough. You need to also make sure that you have the type of lifestyle that will help you lose weight and keep it off. Considering the fact that you are a relatively new mother, it may not really be practical for you to be spending a lot of time at the gym or otherwise carefully following a very detailed diet. However, it really helps if you can do a little bit of exercise every day. This can have a dramatic impact on your ability to lose weight in conjunction with drinking plenty of water and eating reasonable portions.

In the final analysis, women who are interested in losing weight after giving birth to a baby need to take a multidimensional approach to solving the problem. This will include drinking plenty of water, getting some exercise, and eating well. Doing all these things will produce remarkable results.

3. Eat Well

Next, many women who are interested in losing baby fat after giving birth will sometimes make the classic mistake of cutting back on the amount of food that they consume in a manner that is unhealthy. In other words, it can actually be counterproductive to eat dramatically less amounts of food if you are truly interested in losing weight.

The reason why this can be so problematic is because your body will automatically detect that an unusually lower amount of calories are being consumed. This will typically result in a situation whereby your metabolism will slow down. In essence, your body becomes far more efficient at being able to process the calories you do consume and restricts the amount of calories that are burned throughout the day.

What this basically means for a new mother is that she will not experience the type of weight loss she is expecting. By cutting back too much on the amount of food that is being consumed, a woman who has just given birth can not only be potentially affecting the health of her baby -- assuming she is breast-feeding a baby -- but it is also causing a situation whereby her body will not shed as much weight as she thinks it will.

Other downsides associated with restricting the amount of calories you consume include feeling tired, cranky, and not really having the energy to do things. This also includes not really having sufficient amounts of energy to partake in reasonable amounts of exercise that all health experts agree to be very beneficial to losing weight.

The real solution in a situation like this is to make sure that you are eating well. This is not to suggest that you should eat a bunch of junk food or otherwise mistreat yourself by consuming vast quantities of food that really have nothing to do with making sure that you are getting sufficient calories, vitamins, minerals. The idea here is to instead fill yourself with the calories you need but not an excessive amount of calories.

Finally, make sure that you engage in some type of exercise on a regular basis. This can be something as simple as taking walks. What few new mothers realize is that breast-feeding a baby can also help burn up to 800 calories per day. Eat well, do some exercise, and consider breast-feeding your baby. All these things will help you lose much of the extra weight that you accumulated after childbirth.

4. Hot Yoga

I already see the raised eyebrows ! However, did you know that doing hot yoga after pregnancy can not only help improve your psychological outlook, but can really have a lot of positive physical health benefits as well. Some of those positive health benefits that are physical in nature include burning fat and losing weight.

As you may or may not know, bikram yoga -- also known as hot yoga -- is a type of yoga that is typically engaged upon within a very hot environment. More fundamentally, when we talk about yoga we are talking about a series of movements that help the body develop internal calmness which can be really helpful for one's mental outlook while at the same time helping to expand one's strength and flexibility.

When you combine these exercises with an incredibly warm environment -- typically around 95° -- you have a situation where a lot of calories can be burned in a relatively short amount of time. That being said, it's also important to understand that you will need to focus on doing other things that will help you lose the baby fat Some of those other things include making sure that you are eating healthy food. Never try to starve yourself. Your body will detect this and become less likely to shed calories. Actually going into stingy mode.

You also want to make sure that you are doing reasonable amounts of cardiovascular exercise. While it's certainly true that hot yoga will get your heart rate higher -- it is not really a substitute for taking frequent walks that will enable your heart to get some good exercise same time burning a lot of excess calories.

Don't forget that you really need to work on your posture to improve your body image after pregnancy. Bikram yoga is a phenomenal way to not only improve your posture and body image, but it will also really help you reduce the amount of anxiety and stress to you might be experiencing in your life. Giving birth to a baby, while certainly a joyful experience, can also create a lot of anxiety and stress. You owe it to yourself to spend some time focusing on your own health and wellness.

If you have any questions about whether or not you are healthy enough to get involved with any type of yoga activity, be sure to speak your doctor. It only takes a moment, but it helps make sure that you're not doing anything that will harm you.

5. Relax

Finally, far too many women want to try to lose the extra weight that they accumulated during their pregnancy virtually overnight. While it's certainly understandable that a woman would want to look the way she did before her pregnancy began sooner rather than later -- it's important that there be a realistic outlook on this process. After all, it takes approximately 9 months to gain the weight associated with being pregnant. Do you really think it makes sense to assume that most of the baby fat can be lost in nine days or less? Of course not !

Try to really relax and view this process as being something that will take at least two months. The reason why you want to try to view this as a long-term project stems largely from the fact that women who try to lose the weight quickly oftentimes find themselves feeling frustrated and upset by their apparent lack of progress. It's not even a question of them not making progress -- they usually are. But the progress is not fast enough to meet the unrealistic expectations that they have put on themselves. And let us not forget you are also doing this while caring for a newborn.

One of the easiest things that you can do is to set some very basic and realistic goals for yourself. If you do not establish goals, it will be far too easy to simply drift sideways and to assume that you're not really making any progress and to feel more anxious and frustrated about the entire process of losing weight after giving birth. Many medical experts indicate that losing approximately 2 pounds every seven days is reasonable for most women.

When you do the math that works out to losing approximately 16 pounds in two months. While that may not be as much weight as you like to lose, you're giving yourself a realistic benchmark. If you happen to lose more weight than that, great. It should mean that baby fat is melting away ! But try not to stress yourself out over the process.

What many women fail to realize is that they can typically fall victim to something called emotional eating if they find themselves feeling stressed out an anxious over the weight-loss process. No woman wants to find herself in a situation whereby she feel so stressed out and anxious that she does the very thing which will sabotage your efforts -- eating excessive amounts of food.

So as this process is approached, try to relax and realize that it's going to take some time to lose that baby fat.

Chapter 7- Burn Fat and Become Fit with this Basic Routine

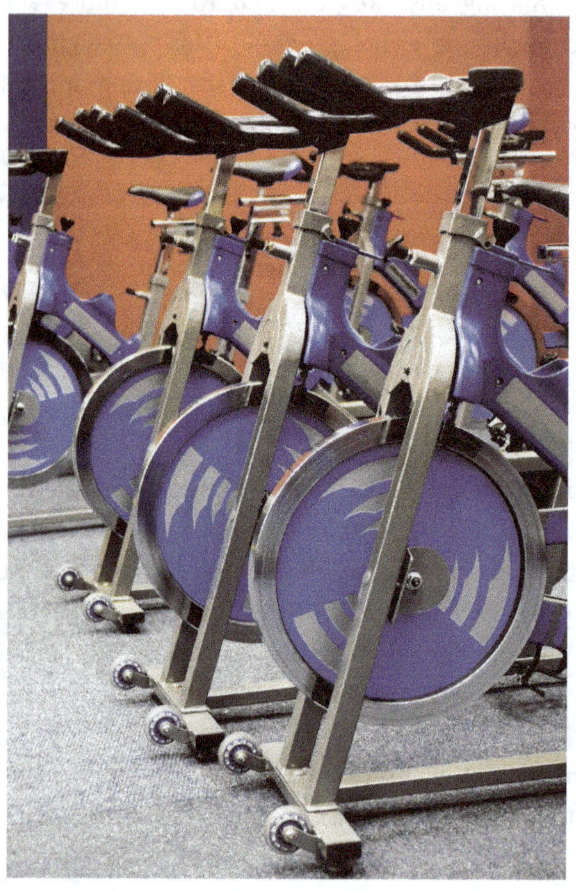

Perform 3 - 5 days a week for maximum results

You can use this as a complete routine in itself or add it on to the end of a cardio session such as a walk or jog. Performed in its entirety, these will get your heart pumping although probably not at the intensity required to keep your cardiovascular system at peak fitness.

If you like, you can preface this routine with a five or ten minute heart rate raiser such as running on the spot, skipping or simply marching fast, knees high and arms pumping.

You can shorten the routine but it is vital you warm up and cool down properly and perform at least two exercises from each section to ensure that all muscle groups have received balanced attention.

Oh and one more thing – remember to have fun!

Warm-Up

Practice the following exercises slowly while concentrating on your breathing pattern.

BREATHING PREPARATION

Lie on your back on a mat or towel, knees bent, feet hip width apart (measure this from the hip bones, not the outer edge of your hips).

Inhale through the nose, exhale through pursed lips. Upon the exhale draw your navel inward and upward and flatten your tummy. Place one hand on your navel if you like to feel your muscles working.

Draw up the pelvic floor muscles gently. If you don't know where these are, the easiest way of describing them is to say that these are the muscles you use when you are trying to hold in a pee! Continue breathing 5-10 times with these muscles pulled in.

Neck and shoulders should stay loose at all times.

LEG LIFTS

These will stabilize your pelvis and provide a foundation for strong abdominal muscles.

Lay your on back, knees bent, hip distance apart. Inhale to prepare – slowly exhale and lift one knee at a time. Keep fingertips on hip bones to check for movement. Press your lower back into the floor slightly as you lower the legs to avoid arching and over working the back. Keep abdominals pulled up and in. Repeat 5 sets.

ABDOMINAL PREPS

These curls prepare you safely for more challenging abdominal exercises. You can either perform them on the floor or on an exercise ball. One thing to remember: never jam your chin into your chest, which results in too much compression of the neck.

Lie on your back either on the floor or across an exercise ball, keeping pelvis and spine neutral, which means neither tucking under with your hips nor arching your lower back away from the floor/ball.

Knees are bent, feet hip-width apart on the floor. To prepare, inhale then exhale.

Cradle the back of your neck in your hands, interweaving your fingers. It is VERY IMPORTANT you do not tug on your neck. Gently curl up, pulling in your stomach, aiming to slide your rib cage toward your pelvis.

Hold for a count of two. Slowly lie back down.

Repeat 5-8 times

KNEELING STRETCH

On hands and knees-line up shoulders with hands and knees under hips. Back is straight and neutral. Inhale to prepare – exhale to draw in abdominals, then without shaking or moving torso slowly reach opposite arm and leg.

Hold for 1 full breath, then return.

Repeat 3-4 sets.

GENTLE BACK EXTENSION

This exercise uses your upper back muscles to lift your head and shoulders off the floor into a gentle back bend instead of pressing up with the arms. Keep your stomach pulled in at all times to protect your lower spine.

Lie on your stomach, keeping pelvis and spine neutral. Legs are straight and together. Elbows are bent, hands by shoulders. To prepare inhale then exhale.

Gently slide shoulder blades down and reach top of head away from tailbone to begin lifting upper back. Allow rib cage to open and maintain bottom ribs in contact with mat.

Hold this position for a count of two and breathe into sides of rib cage without losing your abdominal contraction.

Breathe out and lower upper torso to mat, returning to starting position.

Repeat 5-8 times

REST STRETCH

This exercise stretches your back and abs out the other way, warming up your muscles for the next part of your routine. You can also use it any time to stretch out during your exercise session and it is excellent for general relaxation.

Sit back toward heels, hips lifted, and arms wider than shoulders—hold 5 – 10 deep breaths. For tight lower back/hips, place knees wide apart for comfort.

Ideally, you want to be able to rest your rear on your heels and stretch your arms straight out in front of you, hands flat on the floor.

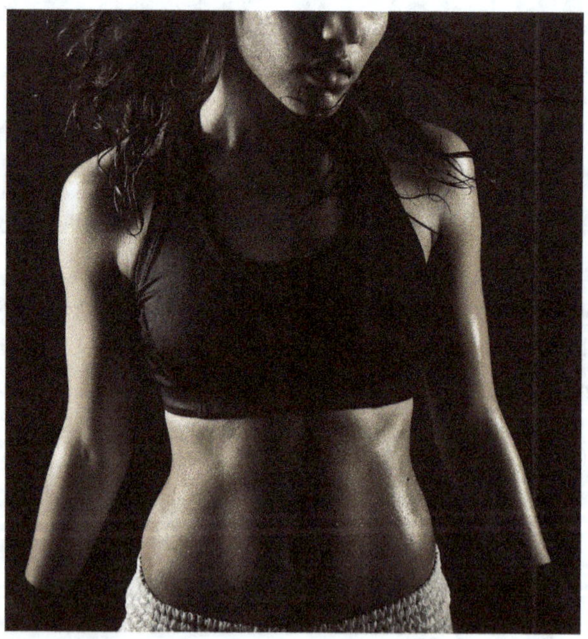

About the Author

John Hamilton is a health enthusiast. He is known as a fat-loss expert, bodybuilder and a nutritionist. Due to his love to stay fit and fat free he has been involved in every aspect of the fitness and weight-loss industry. He has a lot of programs that will ultimately help people to become fit in no time.

Aside from being a nutrition consultant he also manages a fitness gym. He lives in Oklahoma with his wife and children.